ESSENTIAL GUIDE TO DERMATITIS

A Practical Approach to Understanding and Managing Skin Inflammation

DR. CASEY LOREN

1

DISCLAIMER

This book's content is only meant to be used for general informative purposes. Although the author has taken great care to ensure the content is accurate and thorough, no warranties or assurances on the information's accuracy, correctness, or reliability are provided. It is recommended that readers employ their own judgment and discretion when applying any material found in this book to their particular situation.

The information in this book is not intended to replace professional advice, nor is the author an expert in any of the subjects covered. It is recommended that readers consult with experienced professionals regarding any particular issues or concerns.

Any name that may be mentioned or referred in this book does not imply endorsement, recommendation, or relationship on the part of the author with any person, entity, good, website, or association. These references are made only for informational purposes and are not meant to be taken as recommendations or endorsements.

The information contained in this book may cause readers to suffer loss or damage, for which the author disclaims all obligation and accountability. The only people accountable for the decisions and actions taken by readers using the information presented are themselves.

Any names, characters, companies, locations, activities, occasions, and incidents referenced in this book are either made up or the result of the author's imagination. Any likeness to real people, living or dead, or to real things is entirely coincidental.

This book's content may change at any time, without prior notice, according to the author.

The onus is on the reader to verify whether there have been any updates or revisions.

The reader accepts the conditions of this disclaimer by reading this book. Please do not read this book or use its contents if you do not agree to these terms.

Table of Contents

CHAPTER 1

UNDERSTANDING DERMATITIS

Definition and Types of Dermatitis

Dermatitis refers to a group of skin conditions characterized by inflammation, redness, itching, and sometimes blistering or peeling. It can be acute, with sudden onset and short duration, or chronic, lasting for a prolonged period. There are several types of dermatitis, including:

Atopic Dermatitis (Eczema): This is a chronic condition characterized by dry, itchy skin and often runs in families with a history of allergies or asthma.

Contact Dermatitis: This type occurs when the skin comes into contact with an irritant (irritant contact dermatitis) or an allergen (allergic contact dermatitis), leading to a localized reaction.

Seborrheic Dermatitis: This usually affects areas rich in oil glands, such as the scalp, face, and upper chest. It presents with redness, greasy scales, and dandruff-like flakes.

Dyshidrotic Dermatitis: This type results in small blisters on the hands and feet, often triggered by stress, allergies, or exposure to certain metals.

Nummular Dermatitis: Circular or coin-shaped patches of inflamed skin characterize this type, often triggered by dry skin, irritants, or allergies.

Understanding the specific type of dermatitis is crucial for effective management and treatment.

Causes and Triggers

The causes of dermatitis vary depending on the type but may include:

Genetics: Some forms of dermatitis, like atopic dermatitis, have a genetic component.

Immune System Dysfunction: Disorders in the immune system can contribute to the development of dermatitis.

Allergens: Substances like pollen, pet dander, certain foods, or chemicals in skincare products can trigger allergic reactions.

Irritants: Exposure to harsh chemicals, soaps, detergents, or certain fabrics can irritate the skin.

Stress: Emotional stress can exacerbate dermatitis symptoms.

Weather: Extreme temperatures, humidity, or dryness can impact the skin.

Microorganisms: Fungi, bacteria, or viruses can sometimes cause or worsen dermatitis.

Identifying and avoiding triggers is an essential part of managing dermatitis effectively.

Common Symptoms

Symptoms of dermatitis can vary widely but often include:

Itching (pruritus)

Redness (erythema)

Dry, scaly, or cracked skin

Swelling

Blisters or vesicles

Crusting or oozing

Thickened skin (lichenification)

The severity and combination of symptoms depend on the type and extent of dermatitis.

Dermatitis vs. Other Skin Conditions

Dermatitis can be confused with other skin conditions such as psoriasis, rosacea, or fungal infections. However, key differences in symptoms, appearance, and triggers help distinguish dermatitis from these conditions. Proper

diagnosis by a healthcare professional is essential
for accurate treatment.

Diagnosis and Medical Tests

Diagnosing dermatitis typically involves:

Physical Examination: The doctor examines
the skin, asks about symptoms and triggers, and
may inquire about personal or family history of
allergies or skin conditions.

Patch Testing: For suspected contact
dermatitis, patch testing with potential allergens
helps identify specific triggers.

Skin Biopsy: In some cases, a small skin sample
is taken and examined under a microscope to
confirm the diagnosis or rule out other
conditions.

Other tests may be done based on the suspected
type of dermatitis or underlying causes.

Dermatitis in Children and Adults

Dermatitis can affect individuals of all ages. In children, atopic dermatitis (eczema) is common and may improve with age. Adults may develop various types of dermatitis due to occupational exposures, stress, or underlying health conditions. Treatment approaches may differ based on age-related factors and the type of dermatitis.

Impact of Dermatitis on Quality of Life

Dermatitis can significantly impact the quality of life, causing discomfort, sleep disturbances (due to itching), self-consciousness, and interference with daily activities or work. Chronic dermatitis, especially when poorly controlled, can lead to psychological distress and reduced overall well-being.

Global Prevalence and Statistics

The prevalence of dermatitis varies globally, with certain types like atopic dermatitis being more common in developed countries. According to the World Health Organization, atopic dermatitis affects up to 20% of children and 3% of adults worldwide. Contact dermatitis is one of the most prevalent occupational skin diseases, particularly in industries involving chemical exposure.

Historical Perspectives

Historically, dermatitis has been recognized for centuries, with descriptions dating back to ancient medical texts. Early treatments focused on topical remedies, while modern understanding has expanded to include immune mechanisms, genetic factors, and environmental influences.

Current Research and Developments

Ongoing research in dermatitis focuses on:

Understanding genetic and immune factors contributing to different types of dermatitis.

Developing targeted therapies, including biologics and immune modulators.

Exploring the role of the skin microbiome in dermatitis development and management.

Investigating novel topical treatments and formulations for improved symptom control and skin barrier repair.

Advancements in research aim to enhance diagnosis, treatment efficacy, and overall outcomes for individuals with dermatitis.

CHAPTER 2

DERMATITIS: A COMPREHENSIVE OVERVIEW

Anatomy of the Skin:

The skin is our body's largest organ, serving as a protective barrier between our internal organs and the external environment. It consists of three main layers: the epidermis, dermis, and subcutaneous tissue. The epidermis is the outermost layer, providing waterproofing and protection, while the dermis contains blood vessels, nerves, hair follicles, and sweat glands. The subcutaneous tissue houses fat cells that provide insulation and cushioning.

Immunological Basis of Dermatitis:

Dermatitis is often driven by an immune system overreaction to various triggers. Inflammatory responses mediated by immune cells such as T cells, dendritic cells, and cytokines play a crucial role. This immune dysregulation can lead to the characteristic symptoms of dermatitis, including redness, itching, swelling, and skin barrier dysfunction.

Genetic Factors and Predispositions:

Genetics can significantly influence an individual's susceptibility to dermatitis. Certain gene variants may predispose someone to develop specific types of dermatitis, such as atopic dermatitis (eczema) or contact dermatitis. Understanding these genetic factors can help tailor treatment approaches and predict disease outcomes.

Environmental Influences:

Environmental factors like exposure to allergens, irritants, pollutants, humidity levels, and temperature extremes can trigger or exacerbate dermatitis. Occupational exposures, lifestyle choices, and geographical locations can also impact the onset and severity of the condition.

Psychological and Emotional Links:

Psychological stress and emotional factors can influence dermatitis. Stress hormones like cortisol can exacerbate inflammation, while emotional distress may lead to scratching behaviors that worsen skin damage. Addressing these psychological aspects is essential in managing dermatitis effectively.

Role of Allergens and Irritants:

Allergens (e.g., pollen, pet dander, certain foods) and irritants (e.g., harsh chemicals, soaps, detergents) can trigger dermatitis reactions in susceptible individuals. Identifying and avoiding these triggers is key to preventing flare-ups and managing symptoms.

Seasonal Variations in Dermatitis:

Dermatitis symptoms can vary with seasonal changes. For example, cold, dry winter air can exacerbate dry skin and eczema, while hot, humid conditions may worsen sweating and contact dermatitis. Understanding these seasonal patterns helps in implementing appropriate preventive measures.

Associated Health Conditions:

Dermatitis is often associated with other health conditions, such as asthma, allergic rhinitis, autoimmune diseases, and mental health disorders like anxiety and depression. Managing these comorbidities is integral to comprehensive dermatitis care.

Chronic vs. Acute Dermatitis:

Dermatitis can manifest as either acute (short-term) or chronic (long-lasting) conditions. Acute dermatitis may result from direct irritant exposure or allergic reactions and typically resolves with appropriate treatment. Chronic dermatitis, such as atopic dermatitis, requires ongoing management to control symptoms and prevent flare-ups.

Potential Complications and Risks:

Complications of dermatitis can include secondary skin infections, scarring, pigment changes, and psychological impacts like decreased quality of life and social stigma. Long-term scratching can also lead to lichenification (thickening of the skin) and impaired skin barrier function, predisposing to further inflammation and infections. Managing dermatitis promptly and effectively can reduce these risks and improve overall skin health.

CHAPTER 3

TYPES OF DERMATITIS

Atopic Dermatitis (Eczema)

Atopic dermatitis, commonly known as eczema, is a chronic inflammatory skin condition characterized by itchy, red, and dry skin. It often develops during childhood and can persist into adulthood. Genetics, environmental factors, and a compromised skin barrier play significant roles in its development. Common triggers include allergens, irritants, stress, and climate changes. Management involves avoiding triggers, maintaining skin hydration, using emollients, topical corticosteroids for flare-ups, and sometimes systemic medications in severe cases.

Contact Dermatitis (Allergic and Irritant)

Contact dermatitis occurs when the skin comes into contact with substances that trigger an immune response or directly damage the skin.

Allergic contact dermatitis results from exposure to allergens like nickel, fragrances, or latex, leading to an immune reaction. Irritant contact dermatitis occurs due to direct skin damage from substances like soaps, detergents, or chemicals. Both types present with redness, itching, and sometimes blistering. Treatment involves identifying and avoiding triggers, using emollients, topical corticosteroids, and in severe cases, oral medications.

Seborrheic Dermatitis

Seborrheic dermatitis is a common chronic condition characterized by red, scaly patches, typically affecting oily areas like the scalp, face, and chest. It results from a combination of factors including genetics, yeast overgrowth (Malassezia), and an inflammatory response. Symptoms include itching, redness, and flaking skin. Management includes medicated shampoos, topical antifungal agents, corticosteroids, and lifestyle modifications such as stress management and gentle skincare.

Nummular Dermatitis

Nummular dermatitis presents as coin-shaped patches of irritated skin, often triggered by dryness, skin injury, or allergens. It can be intensely itchy and may lead to skin infections if scratched. Treatment involves moisturizing the skin, using topical corticosteroids or calcineurin inhibitors, and identifying and avoiding triggers.

Dyshidrotic Dermatitis

Dyshidrotic dermatitis, also known as pompholyx, manifests as small blisters on the hands and feet, accompanied by itching and redness. The exact cause is unknown, but factors like stress, allergies, and exposure to irritants may contribute. Treatment includes topical corticosteroids, antihistamines for itching, and avoiding triggers like excessive hand washing or allergens.

Stasis Dermatitis

Stasis dermatitis develops in the lower legs due to poor circulation, often seen in individuals with venous insufficiency or varicose veins. Symptoms include swelling, redness, itching, and eventually skin thickening and ulceration. Management focuses on improving circulation, using compression stockings, topical treatments for inflammation, and addressing underlying venous issues.

Neurodermatitis (Lichen Simplex Chronicus)

Neurodermatitis is a skin condition characterized by thick, scaly patches resulting from repeated scratching or rubbing, often due to stress or psychological factors. It commonly affects the neck, wrists, ankles, and genital area. Treatment involves addressing the underlying stressors, using topical corticosteroids, antihistamines for itching, and behavioral therapies to break the itch-scratch cycle.

Perioral Dermatitis

Perioral dermatitis is a facial rash that typically affects the area around the mouth, nose, and eyes. It presents as red, bumpy, and sometimes itchy skin, resembling acne or eczema. The exact cause is unknown but may involve factors like hormonal changes, skincare products, or oral antibiotics. Treatment includes discontinuing potential triggers like steroid creams, using gentle skin care products, topical antibiotics, and sometimes oral medications.

Dermatitis Herpetiformis

Dermatitis herpetiformis is a chronic skin condition associated with celiac disease, characterized by intensely itchy, blistering skin lesions, often on the elbows, knees, and buttocks. It results from an immune reaction to gluten, leading to the deposition of antibodies in the skin. Treatment involves a strict gluten-free diet, dapsone medication to control symptoms, and monitoring for celiac disease complications.

Exfoliative Dermatitis

Exfoliative dermatitis, also called erythroderma, is a severe inflammatory skin disorder characterized by widespread redness, scaling, and shedding of the skin's outer layer. It can result from various underlying conditions such as psoriasis, drug reactions, lymphomas, or autoimmune diseases. Management includes identifying and treating the underlying cause, skin hydration, topical therapies, and in severe cases, hospitalization for supportive care and monitoring.

CHAPTER 4

DERMATITIS TRIGGERS AND RISK FACTORS

Allergens: Pollen, Dust Mites, Pet Dander

Allergens are substances that can trigger an allergic reaction in sensitive individuals. In the case of dermatitis, common allergens include pollen from plants, dust mites commonly found in household dust, and pet dander from animals like cats and dogs. These allergens can come into contact with the skin and cause an immune response, leading to symptoms such as redness, itching, and inflammation. Managing exposure to these allergens through measures like using air purifiers, regular cleaning, and minimizing contact with pets can help reduce dermatitis flare-ups.

Irritants: Soaps, Detergents, Chemicals

Irritants are substances that can directly irritate the skin, leading to dermatitis symptoms. Examples include harsh soaps, detergents, and chemicals found in household products or workplace environments. Prolonged or repeated exposure to these irritants can disrupt the skin's barrier function, causing dryness, redness, and itching. Using gentle, fragrance-free products, wearing protective gloves when handling chemicals, and moisturizing regularly can help protect the skin from irritant-induced dermatitis.

Climate and Weather Conditions

Climate and weather conditions can also influence dermatitis. Dry, cold weather can lead to skin dryness and exacerbate existing dermatitis symptoms, while hot and humid conditions may increase sweat production and potentially trigger flare-ups. Protecting the skin with appropriate clothing, using humidifiers in dry environments, and adjusting skincare routines based on seasonal changes can help manage dermatitis related to climate and weather conditions.

Stress and Emotional Factors

Stress and emotional factors can play a significant role in dermatitis. Stress can weaken the immune system and increase inflammation, making individuals more susceptible to flare-ups. Emotional factors like anxiety, depression, and low self-esteem can also impact dermatitis by affecting skin barrier function and triggering nervous system responses that contribute to skin inflammation. Managing stress through techniques like mindfulness, relaxation exercises, and seeking support from mental health professionals can be beneficial in controlling dermatitis symptoms.

Hormonal Changes

Hormonal changes, such as those occurring during puberty, pregnancy, or menopause, can influence dermatitis. Fluctuations in hormone levels can affect skin oil production, immune responses, and skin barrier function, potentially leading to changes in dermatitis severity. Managing hormonal dermatitis may involve adjusting skincare routines, using hormone-balancing medications under medical guidance, and addressing underlying hormonal imbalances.

Food Allergies and Sensitivities

Certain foods can trigger allergic reactions or sensitivities in susceptible individuals, leading to dermatitis symptoms. Common food allergens include nuts, dairy products, eggs, and shellfish. Identifying and avoiding trigger foods through allergy testing and dietary modifications can help manage dermatitis related to food allergies and sensitivities.

Medications and Topical Treatments

Some medications and topical treatments can cause or exacerbate dermatitis as a side effect. For example, certain antibiotics, antifungals, and acne medications may lead to skin irritation or allergic reactions. It's essential to inform healthcare providers about any known allergies or previous reactions to medications to avoid potential dermatitis flare-ups. Using prescribed medications as directed and following proper skincare routines can also help minimize adverse effects.

Occupational Exposures

Occupational exposures to chemicals, solvents, allergens, and irritants can contribute to occupational dermatitis. Jobs involving frequent handwashing, exposure to cleaning agents, or contact with industrial chemicals increase the risk of developing dermatitis. Employers can implement measures such as providing protective gear, training on the proper handling of hazardous substances, and maintaining a healthy work environment to reduce occupational dermatitis risks.

Genetics and Family History

Genetics and family history play a role in dermatitis susceptibility. Individuals with a family history of allergic conditions like eczema, asthma, or hay fever may be more prone to developing dermatitis themselves. Understanding genetic predispositions can help healthcare providers tailor treatment plans and preventive strategies to manage dermatitis effectively.

Lifestyle Choices and Hygiene Practices

Lifestyle choices and hygiene practices can impact dermatitis. Factors such as smoking, excessive alcohol consumption, poor nutrition, and lack of exercise can affect skin health and overall immune function, potentially worsening dermatitis symptoms. Adopting a healthy lifestyle, including a balanced diet, regular exercise, adequate hydration, and proper skincare habits, can support skin integrity and reduce dermatitis risk factors.

By addressing these triggers and risk factors comprehensively, individuals can better manage dermatitis and improve skin health and quality of life.

CHAPTER 5

MANAGING DERMATITIS: TREATMENT OPTIONS

Topical Corticosteroids:

Topical corticosteroids are a cornerstone in dermatitis management, effectively reducing inflammation and itching. They come in various strengths, from mild to potent, tailored to the severity of the condition and the affected area's sensitivity. It's crucial to follow your dermatologist's guidance on frequency and duration of use to avoid side effects like skin thinning or discoloration.

Moisturizers and Emollients:

Regular use of moisturizers and emollients is vital in dermatitis care to hydrate and strengthen the skin's barrier. Look for products without fragrances or harsh chemicals that can irritate sensitive skin. Applying these after bathing helps lock in moisture, preventing dryness and reducing the risk of flare-ups.

Antihistamines:

Antihistamines are often used to relieve itching associated with dermatitis. They work by blocking histamine receptors, reducing the urge to scratch. Non-sedating antihistamines are preferred for daytime use to avoid drowsiness while sedating ones can be beneficial at night to promote better sleep.

Calcineurin Inhibitors:

Calcineurin inhibitors like tacrolimus and pimecrolimus are prescribed for moderate to severe cases of dermatitis, especially in sensitive areas like the face and groin. They work by suppressing the immune response that leads to inflammation. Long-term use should be monitored closely due to potential side effects.

Phototherapy and Light Therapy:

Phototherapy, including UVB and UVA light treatments, can be effective for certain types of dermatitis, particularly when other treatments haven't provided sufficient relief. It helps reduce inflammation and itching but requires regular sessions under medical supervision to ensure safety and efficacy.

Systemic Medications:

In severe cases, systemic medications like oral corticosteroids or immunosuppressants may be prescribed. These are usually reserved for short-term use due to their potential for side effects, and close monitoring is essential to minimize risks while achieving therapeutic benefits.

Natural and Alternative Remedies:

Some individuals find relief from dermatitis symptoms through natural remedies like oatmeal baths, coconut oil, or herbal extracts with anti-inflammatory properties. However, their effectiveness varies, and it's crucial to consult with a healthcare professional before relying solely on these approaches.

Lifestyle Modifications:

Making lifestyle changes such as avoiding triggers like harsh soaps or allergens, wearing soft clothing, and practicing stress-reducing techniques like meditation or yoga can complement medical treatments and help manage dermatitis symptoms effectively.

Dietary Changes and Supplements:

While there's limited scientific evidence linking specific foods to dermatitis flare-ups, maintaining a balanced diet rich in antioxidants, omega-3 fatty acids, and vitamins can support overall skin health. Supplements like probiotics or fish oil may also be beneficial but should be discussed with a healthcare provider first.

Emerging Therapies and Clinical Trials:

Researchers are continuously exploring new therapies for dermatitis through clinical trials. These may include novel medications, targeted therapies, or biologics that offer hope for improved outcomes, especially for individuals with treatment-resistant forms of the condition. Participating in clinical trials under medical supervision can provide access to cutting-edge treatments and contribute to advancing dermatology knowledge.

CHAPTER 6

PRACTICAL TIPS FOR DERMATITIS CARE

Skincare Routine for Dermatitis:

A well-designed skincare routine is fundamental in managing dermatitis effectively. Begin with gentle, fragrance-free cleansers that won't irritate the skin. Follow up with moisturizers containing ceramides and hyaluronic acid to restore and lock in moisture. Sunscreen is crucial, opt for broad-spectrum SPF 30 or higher to shield against UV rays. Incorporate topical treatments prescribed by your dermatologist as needed, such as corticosteroids or calcineurin inhibitors.

Clothing and Fabric Choices:

Choosing the right clothing can significantly impact dermatitis management. Opt for loose-fitting, breathable fabrics like cotton to minimize friction and allow the skin to breathe. Avoid harsh materials like wool or synthetic fibers that can exacerbate irritation. Wash clothes with mild, hypoallergenic detergents and skip fabric softeners or dryer sheets that may contain irritants.

Home Environment Adjustments:

Create a skin-friendly home environment by maintaining optimal humidity levels with a humidifier, especially during dry seasons. Use gentle, non-irritating cleaning products for surfaces and laundry. Keep pets groomed to reduce exposure to dander and allergens. Consider air purifiers to filter out airborne pollutants that can trigger dermatitis flare-ups.

Managing Stress and Emotional Well-being:

Stress can worsen dermatitis symptoms, so prioritize stress management techniques like mindfulness, meditation, or yoga. Engage in activities that promote relaxation and positive emotions. Seek support from friends, family, or a therapist if needed to cope with the emotional challenges associated with chronic skin conditions.

Allergen Avoidance Strategies:

Identify and avoid allergens that trigger dermatitis flare-ups. This may include certain foods, pollen, pet dander, or specific skincare products. Keep a diary to track potential triggers and modify your environment accordingly. Consult an allergist for comprehensive allergy testing if necessary.

Proper Bathing and Hygiene Practices:

Practice gentle bathing and hygiene routines to prevent skin irritation. Use lukewarm water instead of hot water, limit bathing time, and avoid harsh soaps or exfoliants. Pat your skin dry gently with a soft towel and apply moisturizer immediately after bathing to lock in moisture.

Recognizing Flare-Up Triggers:

Learn to recognize and avoid triggers that can lead to dermatitis flare-ups. Common triggers include stress, certain foods, environmental factors like pollen or pollution, and contact with irritants like harsh chemicals or fabrics. Keep a symptom diary to track patterns and identify potential triggers.

Traveling with Dermatitis:

Plan when traveling with dermatitis to minimize flare-up risks. Pack travel-sized skincare products to maintain your routine. Research local climate and allergen levels at your destination. Carry medications or prescriptions as needed and consider travel insurance for medical emergencies.

Working with Healthcare Providers:

Establish a collaborative relationship with dermatologists and healthcare providers. Follow their treatment plans diligently, attend regular check-ups, and communicate any concerns or changes in symptoms promptly. Be proactive in discussing treatment options and lifestyle adjustments to optimize dermatitis management.

Support Systems and Communities:

Seek support from dermatitis support groups or online communities to connect with others facing similar challenges. Share experiences, tips, and resources for coping with dermatitis. Consider joining patient advocacy organizations for access to educational materials and advocacy opportunities.

CHAPTER 7
DERMATITIS IN SPECIAL POPULATIONS

Pediatric Dermatitis:

Infants and Children Dermatitis in children can be challenging due to their delicate skin and unique reactions to environmental factors. Understanding the causes and triggers is crucial for effective management. Common types include atopic dermatitis (eczema), contact dermatitis, and seborrheic dermatitis. Treatments often involve gentle skincare, moisturizers, avoiding irritants, and in some cases, topical medications prescribed by a healthcare professional.

Dermatitis in Adolescents and Teens Adolescents and teens may experience dermatitis due to hormonal changes, increased stress levels, and lifestyle factors. Acne, eczema, and contact dermatitis are frequent concerns. Treatment plans often include a combination of skincare routines, stress management techniques, dietary adjustments, and medication if necessary. Education about proper skin care habits is essential during this developmental stage.

Adult-Onset Dermatitis

Adult-onset dermatitis can arise from various causes such as stress, environmental exposures, hormonal changes, and genetic predispositions. Conditions like eczema, psoriasis, and allergic reactions become more prevalent in adulthood. Treatment focuses on identifying triggers, adopting suitable skincare regimens, managing stress, and sometimes using prescription medications or therapies like phototherapy.

Dermatitis in the Elderly

The elderly population is susceptible to dermatitis due to age-related changes in skin structure, decreased immune function, and medical conditions like diabetes or vascular disorders. Common concerns include dry skin, eczema, and contact dermatitis. Management involves gentle skincare, moisturizing products, regular skin checks, and addressing underlying health issues that may contribute to dermatitis.

Pregnancy and Dermatitis Management

Pregnancy can affect dermatitis in various ways, with hormonal shifts influencing skin conditions like eczema or psoriasis. Certain treatments may not be suitable during pregnancy, necessitating careful management. Emollients, mild topical steroids, and antihistamines are commonly used with medical supervision. Communication between dermatologists and obstetricians is vital for safe and effective care.

Dermatitis in Athletes and Active Individuals

Athletes and active individuals face unique challenges with dermatitis due to increased sweat, friction, and exposure to sports equipment or environmental factors. Conditions like frictional dermatitis, athlete's foot, and allergic reactions to equipment are common. Prevention involves proper hygiene, breathable clothing, moisture-wicking fabrics, and prompt treatment of any skin issues to prevent infections.

Occupational Dermatitis Challenges

Occupational dermatitis occurs due to exposure to irritants or allergens in the workplace, such as chemicals, solvents, or frequent handwashing. Common forms include irritant contact dermatitis and occupational eczema. Prevention strategies include protective clothing, gloves, barrier creams, regular skin assessments, and workplace education on skin safety practices.

Dermatitis and Mental Health

Dermatitis can have a significant impact on mental health, leading to stress, anxiety, and reduced quality of life. Chronic conditions like eczema or psoriasis may cause emotional distress and affect self-esteem. Managing dermatitis involves addressing mental health concerns through counseling, stress reduction techniques, support groups, and holistic approaches to well-being.

Cultural and Ethnic Considerations

Cultural and ethnic factors can influence dermatitis presentation, management practices, and perceptions of skincare. Skin types, beauty standards, traditional remedies, and cultural practices may impact how individuals experience and manage dermatitis. Healthcare providers should consider these factors when developing personalized treatment plans and providing patient education.

Dermatitis in Individuals with Disabilities

Individuals with disabilities may face specific challenges with dermatitis management due to mobility limitations, sensory issues, or healthcare access barriers. Caregivers play a crucial role in skincare routines, recognizing symptoms, and seeking appropriate medical care. Tailored approaches considering the individual's needs, abilities, and communication methods are essential for effective dermatitis management.

Understanding and addressing dermatitis in special populations requires a comprehensive approach that considers biological, psychological, social, and cultural factors. Collaboration between healthcare providers, patients, caregivers, and relevant support networks is key to achieving optimal outcomes and improving quality of life.

CHAPTER 8

PREVENTING DERMATITIS: STRATEGIES AND PRECAUTIONS

Skin Barrier Protection

Effective skin barrier protection is crucial in preventing dermatitis. This involves using appropriate skincare products that are gentle on the skin, maintaining proper hydration levels, and avoiding harsh chemicals or irritants. Barrier creams and ointments can also be beneficial, especially for individuals in occupations with high exposure to irritants or allergens.

Hygiene Best Practices

Maintaining good hygiene practices is essential for preventing dermatitis. This includes regular handwashing with mild soap and water, avoiding excessive use of hand sanitizers that can dry out the skin, and using moisturizers to keep the skin hydrated. It's also important to use clean, non-irritating clothing and bedding materials.

Early Intervention and Education

Early intervention plays a key role in preventing dermatitis from worsening. Educating individuals about the early signs and symptoms of dermatitis, such as redness, itching, and dryness, can help them seek timely medical advice and treatment. Dermatologists and healthcare providers can provide valuable guidance on preventive measures and suitable skincare routines.

Environmental Control Measures

Controlling environmental factors is crucial for preventing dermatitis. This includes minimizing exposure to known irritants or allergens, such as chemicals, detergents, and certain fabrics. Creating a clean and allergen-free environment, especially in workplaces or homes, can significantly reduce the risk of dermatitis.

Allergen Testing and Avoidance

Identifying specific allergens through testing, such as patch testing or blood tests, can guide individuals in avoiding triggers that can exacerbate dermatitis. This may involve avoiding certain foods, plants, or substances that cause allergic reactions and implementing strict avoidance measures in daily routines.

Lifestyle Modifications for Prevention

Making lifestyle modifications can greatly contribute to preventing dermatitis. This includes adopting a healthy diet rich in antioxidants and omega-3 fatty acids, managing stress levels, getting adequate sleep, and avoiding habits like smoking that can negatively impact skin health. Regular exercise can also improve overall well-being and skin resilience.

Public Health Initiatives

Public health initiatives are essential for raising awareness about dermatitis prevention. This can include providing educational resources, organizing workshops or seminars, and collaborating with healthcare professionals to promote preventive measures at the community level. Public health campaigns can also advocate for policies that support skin health and safety.

Dermatitis Awareness Campaigns

Dermatitis awareness campaigns play a vital role in educating the public about the importance of skin health and prevention strategies. These campaigns can use various platforms such as social media, posters, and informational materials to reach a wide audience. Emphasizing the impact of dermatitis on quality of life and highlighting preventive measures can encourage proactive skin care practices.

Workplace Safety and Regulations

Ensuring workplace safety and adherence to regulations is crucial for preventing occupational dermatitis. Employers should provide proper training on skin protection, offer suitable personal protective equipment (PPE), and implement measures to minimize exposure to harmful substances. Regular monitoring and risk assessments can help identify and address potential hazards in the workplace.

Advocacy and Policy Recommendations

Advocacy efforts and policy recommendations are instrumental in promoting dermatitis prevention on a larger scale. Advocacy groups, healthcare organizations, and policymakers can work together to develop and implement policies that prioritize skin health, support research on preventive measures, and ensure access to quality dermatological care. Engaging stakeholders and advocating for proactive initiatives can lead to meaningful changes in public health approaches to dermatitis prevention.

CHAPTER 9
LIVING WITH DERMATITIS: COPING AND THRIVING

Psychological Impact of Dermatitis

Living with dermatitis can have a significant psychological impact on individuals. The constant itching, discomfort, and visible symptoms can lead to feelings of frustration, embarrassment, and even depression or anxiety in some cases. It's crucial to acknowledge and address these emotional aspects as part of holistic dermatitis management.

Coping Strategies and Resilience Building

Effective coping strategies are essential for managing dermatitis. These can include stress-reduction techniques like mindfulness, deep breathing exercises, and relaxation therapies.

Building resilience involves developing a positive mindset, cultivating adaptability, and seeking support from healthcare professionals, support groups, or therapists when needed.

Supportive Relationships and Communication

Having supportive relationships and open communication channels with family, friends, and healthcare providers is vital. It allows individuals with dermatitis to express their feelings, seek help when necessary, and receive understanding and encouragement from their support network.

Dermatitis and Self-Esteem

Dermatitis can impact self-esteem due to visible symptoms and the challenges it presents in daily life. Building self-esteem involves focusing on personal strengths, practicing self-care, and seeking professional help or counseling if self-esteem issues become significant.

Setting Realistic Goals and Expectations

Setting realistic goals and expectations is crucial in managing dermatitis effectively. This includes understanding limitations, prioritizing self-care, and working with healthcare professionals to develop achievable treatment plans and lifestyle adjustments.

Finding Joy and Fulfillment

Despite the challenges of dermatitis, finding joy and fulfillment in life is possible. Engaging in activities that bring happiness, connecting with loved ones, practicing gratitude, and focusing on positive experiences can contribute to overall well-being.

Overcoming Stigma and Misconceptions

Overcoming stigma and misconceptions associated with dermatitis involves education, advocacy, and promoting awareness. Encouraging open discussions, challenging stereotypes, and sharing personal experiences can help reduce stigma and improve understanding.

Pursuing Hobbies and Interests

Engaging in hobbies and interests is beneficial for mental well-being and can provide a welcome distraction from dermatitis symptoms. Whether it's art, music, sports, or other activities, pursuing passions can enhance the quality of life.

Advocacy and Community Engagement

Advocacy and community engagement play crucial roles in raising awareness, promoting research, and improving resources for dermatitis. Getting involved in advocacy groups, participating in awareness campaigns, and sharing experiences can contribute to positive change.

Celebrating Personal Triumphs

Celebrating personal triumphs, no matter how small, is important in the journey of living with dermatitis. Recognizing achievements, overcoming challenges, and acknowledging progress can boost confidence and motivation.

Overall, living with dermatitis involves a holistic approach that addresses physical symptoms, emotional well-being, and social support. By implementing coping strategies, fostering resilience, building supportive relationships, and embracing life's joys and challenges, individuals can thrive despite the condition.

CHAPTER 10

THE FUTURE OF DERMATITIS RESEARCH AND CARE

Innovations in Dermatitis Treatment:

The future of dermatitis treatment is marked by remarkable innovations that promise more effective and tailored solutions for patients. Researchers are delving into novel therapeutic avenues such as biologics, targeted immunomodulators, and advanced topical formulations. These innovations aim to not only alleviate symptoms but also target the underlying causes of dermatitis, leading to better long-term outcomes and improved quality of life for patients.

Precision Medicine Approaches:

Precision medicine in dermatitis heralds a paradigm shift in treatment strategies. By leveraging genetic, environmental, and lifestyle factors, clinicians can tailor therapies to individual patients, optimizing efficacy and minimizing side effects. This personalized approach holds immense promise in identifying precise triggers and mechanisms of dermatitis, paving the way for more targeted interventions and improved patient outcomes.

Genetics and Personalized Therapies:

Advancements in genomic research have unveiled crucial insights into the genetic basis of dermatitis. Understanding the interplay of genetic factors in disease pathogenesis enables the development of personalized therapies tailored to an individual's genetic profile. From pharmacogenomics to gene editing technologies, the future holds immense potential for precise, gene-based interventions in dermatitis management.

Biomarkers and Diagnostic Advancements:

Biomarkers play a pivotal role in revolutionizing dermatitis diagnosis and management. Emerging biomarker technologies, including transcriptomics, proteomics, and metabolomics, enable early disease detection, subtype classification, and treatment response prediction. These diagnostic advancements not only enhance clinical decision-making but also facilitate personalized therapeutic strategies based on individual biomarker profiles.

Technology in Dermatitis Management:

The integration of technology, such as telemedicine, wearable sensors, and artificial intelligence, is reshaping dermatitis management. Telemedicine platforms facilitate remote consultations, monitoring, and treatment adjustments, improving access to care and patient convenience. Additionally, AI-driven algorithms aid in diagnosis, treatment planning, and predictive analytics, optimizing therapeutic outcomes and reducing healthcare disparities.

Global Collaboration and Initiatives:

Global collaboration and initiatives are pivotal in advancing dermatitis research and care. Collaborative efforts among researchers, clinicians, industry stakeholders, and patient advocacy groups foster knowledge sharing, resource allocation, and coordinated research endeavors. International initiatives promote standardization of diagnostic criteria, treatment guidelines, and patient education, ensuring equitable access to high-quality dermatitis care worldwide.

Patient-Centered Care Models:

The future of dermatitis care embraces patient-centered models that prioritize individual needs, preferences, and experiences. Shared decision-making, patient education, and holistic support systems empower patients to actively participate in their care journey. Tailored care plans, psychosocial interventions, and patient-reported outcomes measures enhance treatment adherence, satisfaction, and overall well-being.

Improving Access to Dermatitis Care:

Efforts to improve access to dermatitis care encompass diverse strategies, including telemedicine expansion, community outreach programs, and healthcare policy reforms. Leveraging digital health technologies, training non-specialist providers, and implementing multidisciplinary care models bridge geographical, socioeconomic, and cultural barriers, ensuring equitable access to timely and comprehensive dermatitis care for all patients.

Addressing Environmental Factors:

Environmental factors play a pivotal role in dermatitis development and exacerbation. Future research and interventions focus on identifying environmental triggers, such as allergens, pollutants, and climate-related factors, and implementing targeted mitigation strategies. Environmental modifications, lifestyle interventions, and public health initiatives aim to create dermatitis-friendly environments, reducing disease burden and improving outcomes.

Hope and Progress in Dermatitis Research:

The landscape of dermatitis research is characterized by a sense of hope and progress fueled by scientific breakthroughs, collaborative efforts, and patient advocacy. Ongoing research endeavors, including clinical trials, translational studies, and basic science investigations, promise novel therapeutic targets, diagnostic tools, and preventive strategies. With a growing understanding of disease mechanisms and a collective commitment to innovation, the future holds immense promise for advancing dermatitis research and transforming patient care.

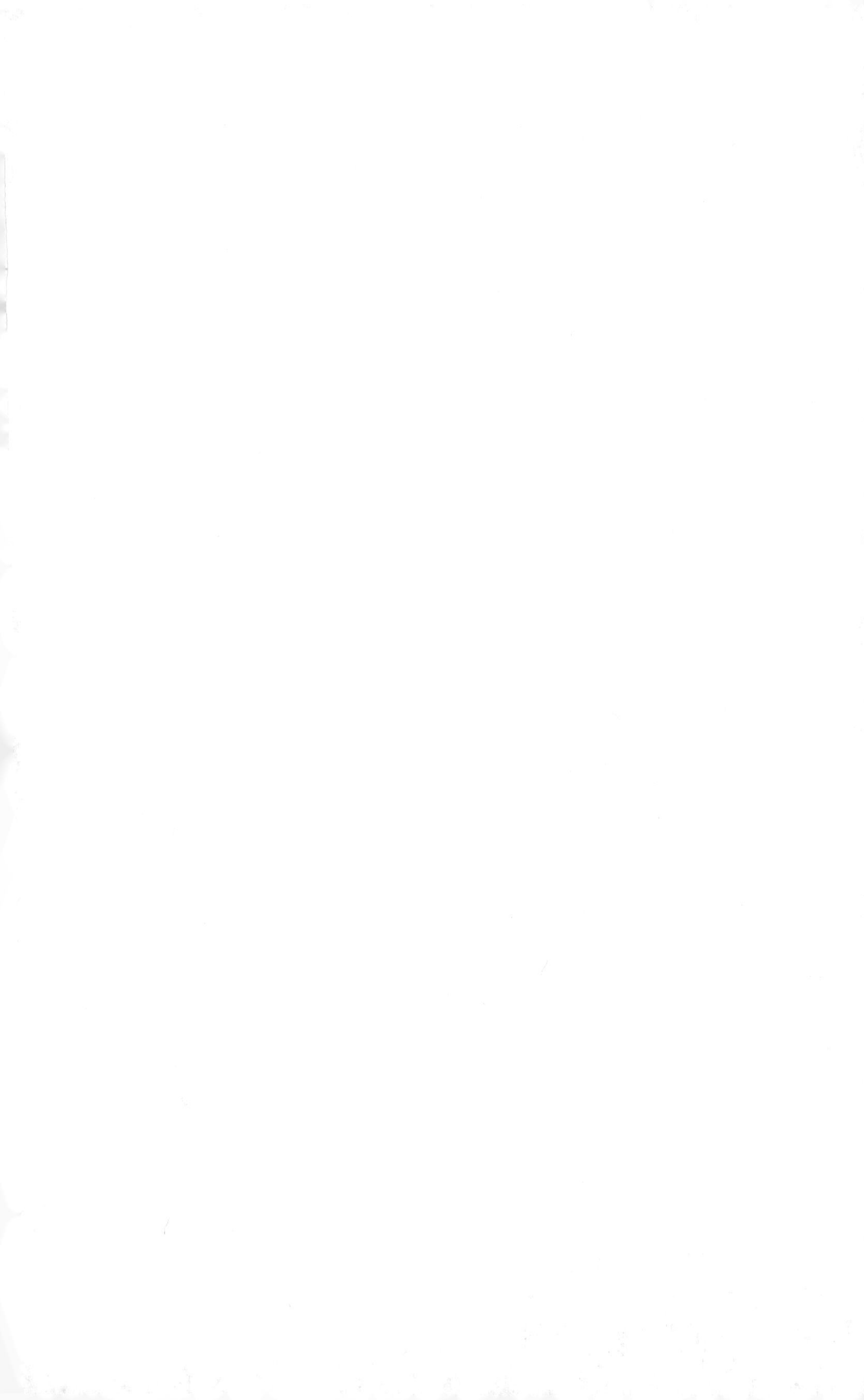